Low Carb Diet For Weight Loss Secrets

How To Effortlessly Lose Weight Fast With The Low Carb Diet

Matthew Jones

Table of Contents

Introduction

I want to thank you and congratulate you for downloading the book, *"Low Carb Diet For Weight Loss Secrets-How To Effortlessly Lose Weight With The Low Carb Diet"*.

This book expounds on the low carb diet and introduces several weight loss secrets as well as strategies and tips on how to successfully implement the low carb diet in your life.

There is a high chance that you've already tried a ton of different diet plans and weight loss strategies that simply didn't lead to the desired weight loss effect, or you just lost the weight only to gain it all back. Chances are you've tried your best, but the techniques simply didn't work. If this is the case, you don't have to worry. This book will not only give you the information you need to know about the low carb diet and its amazing benefits but also provide you with a few easy strategies and tips on how to effortlessly get rid of the few excess pounds.

You will be happy to know, that the low carb diet is quite different from other diets. It has been proven by various scientific sources that the low carb diet is extremely beneficial to your health. However, this is not even the best part. What's great about the low carb diet is that it requires little to no excess work. Don't think that there aren't challenges that arise from the implementation of the low carb diet. As with any other diet or life-changing plan, you will have to face certain restrictions, which may be a bit too much for your willpower. However, this book will provide you with a few low carb diet weight loss secrets, tips and strategies to help you easily deal with any challenge that arises from the restrictions of the diet.

What Is The Low Carb Diet?

If you have chosen the low carb diet, you are already on the right path to effortless weight loss. The low carb diet is not only a great way to get rid of the excess pounds, but also has many health benefits. However, what exactly is the low carb diet?

Carbohydrates in food are the prime source of energy for our bodies. They perform numerous roles in our bodies, including the storage of energy, improving our immune system and more. They are an important part of our nutrition, but are also the prime factor for excess fat and obesity. Why?

Most of the foods that we love to eat have high quantities of carbohydrates. While it is important for our body to have energy, we only manage to use a small portion of the energy that we get from the carbohydrates. The rest of the energy is conserved in the body in form of fat.

The low carb diet is concentrated on lowering carbohydrate intake, without you having to face a lot of restrictions and challenges. Generally used to lose weight effortlessly, the diet has several health benefits. For instance, it reduces the risk factors associated with diabetes, cancer, heart disease and more.

Moreover, as there are only a few challenges that you will have to face if you implement the low crab diet in your life, you will not only be getting slimmer, but will also be:

i. Enjoying various amounts of different foods.

ii. Changing Your Eating Habits for the Better.

iii. Strengthening your Immune System.

Does It Work?

As aforementioned, carbohydrates are our bodies' main source of fuel. Carbohydrates are classified into two categories namely sugars and starches, which fuel every activity you are involved in. It seems unnatural that lowering your carbohydrate intake, as the low carb diet suggests, will help you lose weight while gaining health benefits. However, it is true.

When our carbohydrate intake is too high, most of the carbohydrates in our body are directly converted into excess fat. They also trigger the production of more insulin, the fat storing hormone. The more carbohydrates are in your body, the more glucose is in your blood thus the more insulin is produced. This leads to serious diseases such as heart disease and diabetes and prevents the fat breakdown in your body.

The low carb diet truly does works. However, what is best about it is that you have one of the widest varieties of foods available for you to eat. Therefore, if you don't like monotonous meals every day, you will love the low carb diet. As with any diet, there are restrictions and you will have to face certain challenges that will test your will power. The fact still remains that the low carb diet is definitely one of the easiest and effortless ways to achieve weight loss.

Top 5 Weight Loss Secrets

Before delving more into the low carb diet, it would be important for you to know some weight loss secrets that will make it easier for you to face the challenges that come with adopting any diet including the low carb diet.

Secret #1: Exercise Is Great and Does Not Always Require Effort

Even though the low carb diet will help you get rid of your excess pounds rather quickly, the process still needs time. However, if you combine the diet with regular exercise, you will be able to see results much more quickly. One of the things you should be aware of is that exercise does not always require effort. If you have no time or simply do not want to go to the gym or jog in the park, don't worry; there is a ton of other ways to get your body to burn fat. One of the best ways is through yoga, Pilates or dancing. But you know what's even better? Sex! That's right; don't be scared to get frisky, as it will help you get rid of excess fat even faster.

Secret #2: Dieting Can be Rather Fun

What most people don't take into account is the positive sides of diets that come on top of the health benefits and the weight loss. When talking about the low carb diet, you'd be surprised by the variety of foods available that you did not even know existed simply by concentrating more on your carbohydrates. Start this diet with the enthusiasm that you will get to eat new foods and tasty meals without necessarily having to take carbohydrates.

Secret #3: It's All About the Mindset

It is scientifically proven that your mindset has an effect on your performance when starting any action. If you think of the diet as a positive new thing for you, then you will have no problem with starting the low carb diet. Moreover, if you keep your mindset about the diet in the positive scale, you will be seeing the weight loss benefits much faster.

Secret #4: Get your Sleep Schedule Right

One of the most important factors that are overlooked by many is sleep. Although, people don't tend to stress on the importance of a healthy sleep schedule in diets, sleep is a vital part of your weight loss even when you talk of the essence of exercise. Sleep helps the body regenerate, while keeping everything in check. If you want your diet to be successful, get enough sleep.

Secret #5: Be Careful Who You Tell

Have you tried dieting before? Have you told the people who are closest to you what you will be doing? Did they make jokes? If the answer is yes, don't worry. It is common that the people who are closest to you will make jokes and statements regarding your success or failure. It is almost certain that they don't want to harm you in any way, but the truth is, they do. Each statement or a joke has a negative impact on both your conscious and subconscious mind. Make sure not to tell many people when dieting, as it will definitely be easier for you if you keep it to yourself at first. Share with people your plan once you feel confident enough that you are going to succeed with it. Telling people who are likely to support you will also give you the morale to go on. Actually, you will have a stronger drive since you will not want to let down these people.

Successful Strategies To Implement The Low Carb Diet In Your Life

As mentioned in the previous chapter, you need to be aware of different weight loss secrets when going on a low carb diet. However, knowing that you want to go on a low carb diet and actually doing it are completely different things. Here are a few basic successful strategies you can use based on your character description in order to implement the low carb diet in your life easily.

Would You Describe Yourself As Addicted To Unhealthy Food?

One of the worst cases is when you want to implement a diet in your life when you are addicted to unhealthy food. If this is the case for you, make sure to concentrate on your willpower as much as possible. However, don't stress out and don't worry. The easiest way to get rid of an addiction is to replace it with another good habit; something you equally love but is not harmful.

Just as smokers quit cigarettes by chewing gum, try to replace your addiction to unhealthy food with a healthy one. This may seem impossible, but it is far easier to do. Once you have chosen to implement the low carb diet in your life, you will have a ton of tasty options of food to choose from. Every time you think of unhealthy food, simply head to the cupboard and get some almonds or drink a glass of water until you feel that your hunger is tamed.

This strategy works well in taming food addiction. Remember, you are not addicted to the unhealthy food as much as you are addicted to the habit of eating it. If you replace the habit with eating more healthy food, it will be far easier to you to implement the low carb diet in your life.

Do You Have Problems With Your Willpower And Self-Discipline?

If you experience more trouble with your willpower and the self-discipline part of the implementation of the diet rather than the food itself, you can try implementing different tips and tricks that will help you out on your path to successful weight loss.

One of the best tips, as mentioned before is keeping a positive mindset. Rather than perceiving the diet as something that you "must" or "have to" do, choose to view it as something that you "choose to" do. Make sure to always have conversations with yourself. Even though this may sound far-fetched, it is extremely helpful.

For example, every time you hear your inner voice telling you that you "can't continue" doing the diet. Ask yourself "why?" Ask yourself further questions, such as "why did I choose to undertake this diet in the first place?" Self-talk is helpful regarding any issue connected with self-discipline and is an extremely helpful strategy to keep in mind when implementing the low carb diet.

Another thing you might try is to separate your food and snacks in portions. Make sure to keep a few portions of your meal, the portions being not bigger than two of your fists, in your fridge. Separate your snacks into portions as well. When starting to eat, take one of the portions. When finished eating, even if you go to the fridge for a second one, you will most probably never go for a third. This will help you out a lot, as you will be able to have more time to talk and ask yourself the valuable questions, when going to get that next meal. This will help you eat relatively less than you usually do; you will be surprised as to how helpful it actually is.

Are You A More Imaginative Person?

If you describe yourself as an imaginative person, then make sure to use this to your advantage when implementing the low carb diet. Your mindset is truly a powerful thing and if you are quite imaginative, you should always try to visualize the diet as something amazing. Whether you will envision the diet as a fun new experience or a vicious challenge that you have to complete in order for you to be a better person is totally up to you. However, make sure that the said vision of the diet will be most beneficial to you.

Effortless Weight Loss

After you've familiarized yourself with the basics of the low carb diet and the successful strategies, secrets and tips that you have to know in order to successfully implement the diet in your life, it is time to learn why it is effortless. The answer to the question is rather simple – the diet requires little to no effort because you have a wide variety of foods to eat. How exactly do you choose your food and which foods you should avoid? Which are the most common foods with high quantities of carbohydrates?

The basic foods that you shall eat include:

Meat
Fish
Eggs
Vegetables
Fruits
Nuts
Seeds
High-Fat Dairy
Healthy Fats & Oils

The basic foods that you shall not eat include:

Sugar
Wheat
Seed Oils
Artificial Sweeteners
Low-Fat Products
Highly Processed "Diet" and Low-Fat Food

The general consumption of sugar is probably the most difficult to avoid, but if you implement the strategies mentioned in the previous chapters in the book, you will find it far easier to start your low carb diet.

Need a more detailed list of foods to avoid? Here's a quick one:

Sugar is contained in many things, but you most generally should avoid fruit juices, agave, ice cream, cakes, soft drinks, and many others.

Gluten Grains: Any type of bread, wheat products, spelt, pastas and more.

"Low-Fat" Products: Generally, any product that is labeled as "diet" or "low-fat" is highly processed; thus, it is very unhealthy for you to eat especially due to its high carbohydrate quantities

Other Highly Processed Foods: Anything that is processed is not recommended

High Omega-6-Seed and Vegetable oils: Though oils are considered good in some cases, any vegetable oil should be avoided in the low carb diet

Trans Fats: Especially "Hydrogenated" or "partially hydrogenated" oils should also be avoided.

As you have noticed, you don't have to avoid that many food choices. Probably, the hardest one to avoid is the sugar, as it is found in almost everything. However, make sure to give it your best to avoid it in order to achieve fast and effortless weight loss via the low carb diet. You may consider using honey or any other natural sweetener that may not contain as much calories (this should definitely controlled).

If you want to be more exact in the numbers as to what your carbohydrate intake should be, make sure to focus to a maximum of 50 to 150 grams per day. However, be sure to aim at more healthy carbohydrate choices and avoid sugars.

Low Carb Diet Tips And Suggestions

By now, you should be familiar with almost everything needed for you to implement the low carb diet in your life. However, it is not always as easy as it sounds. For some, the "all or nothing" approach may be beneficial, but in most cases, people fail after the first few weeks or even days. If you want to truly succeed, you should be in for the long haul.

Start making small changes in your diet. For example, in the first few days, change only one of your meals to be a low carb one then go with two and after two-three weeks, make sure to follow the rules of the low carb diet fully. This does not grant an instant result, but it is an effortless weight loss method. Additionally, this will definitely change your eating habits for the better.

Keeping track of your progress is also an essential part of the low carb diet. Once you have replaced all of your meals with low carb meals, make sure to start keeping track of your progress. However, don't only trust the scale and what it shows. Make sure to take regular pictures of your body every week for your own personal assessment. Usually, the first results of the low carb diet can be noticed within three weeks of the official start of your low carb diet.

The first month of the diet is the hardest mainly because the results are not visibly noticeable. However, once you reach the one-month mark, be rest assured that you will visibly be getting thinner every single week. Make sure to keep your positive mindset at all times.

Even if you 'fail' midway the diet by eating something that you should avoid, don't quit and mark that as a failure, but rather continue with the diet. One of the biggest mistakes you can make is to consider your diet a failure when you eat one meal that is not included in the diet plan. However, you may tend to slack off a bit. That being said, one meal out of the diet every now and then won't be a huge issue but you should always try to avoid it. Make sure not to give yourself excuses but rather act more, keep a positive mindset and remind yourself why and how the low carb diet will help you out.

Another common mistake you can make when on a low carb diet is to think that a healthy eating habit requires a big budget. This is not necessarily the case with the low carb diet. What I love more about the low carb diet is that you will actually be spending less money for food, which is far healthier for you and will lead you to effortless weight loss.

Getting From Thinking And Planning To Doing

Once you have created a diet plan like the one given in the chapter above, you should get from thinking and planning to actually doing. This is the most important part of the process and a point at which many people fail. Once you are ready to start, don't give yourself excuses and just get going. Rather than setting a date, or a day of the month, simply start the change today. You will see that once you start, everything becomes far easier.

At this point, you should already be ready mentally to start your diet. All you have to do is act. If you don't have the time to create a detailed meal plan, don't worry. Just make sure that you get rid of all food that you should avoid and buy food that you should eat in the low carb diet.

It may sound extreme, but if you are ready to start the diet and are confident in yourself, simply get up and clean your fridge and cupboards from everything that you should avoid. Give it to a friend or a neighbor, because if there is no such food within your reach, the chances that you will fail in your diet are greatly reduced. We are all human and at the end of the day, when something is right in front of us, regardless of our willpower, we may not be able to avoid it. So make sure to get rid of food that you should avoid. Go to the market and buy food that you truly need to implement into your diet plan.

Don't know what exactly to buy? Here's a short list of items:

Eggs
Cottage Cheese
Tuna (without additional oils)
Any fruits or vegetables that you like

Soybeans
Meat (Chicken, beef, fish)
Turkey slices
Dressings and Spices (such as the fat free thousand island dressing)
Crackers
Almonds
Any Type of Nuts

Once your home is full of low carb food, it will be far easier for you to actually implement your diet. Beware, as the first two weeks are probably the most important ones in your path to weight loss. However, once you get in the habit of eating right, you will be left surprised as to how easy it actually is to lose weight and have the lean body that you've always wanted.

Give yourself time and don't be stressed. Big changes in your life require time and nothing can happen in an instant. However, every day you will be getting closer and closer to a change for the better. Once again, make sure to keep that in mind and remind yourself why you have chosen the low carb diet.

Low Carb Diet Recipes
To Get You Started

This book would not be complete without a few recipes to get you started on your journey to losing weight with the low carb diet. Below are several recipes you can try out.

Low Carb Breakfast recipes

Almond Strawberry smoothie

Ingredients

16 oz. unsweetened almond milk

¼ cup frozen strawberries

4 oz. heavy cream

1 tsp vanilla extract

½ tsp artificial sweetener

Instructions

Put all ingredients in your blender and blend until smooth. Add a little water to thin it down.

Serves 1.

Low Carb Breakfast Meatballs

Ingredients

   1 lb lean ground beef

   2 tbsp onion, minced

   32 oz. pork sausage

   ½ lb shredded cheddar cheese

   Ground black pepper to taste

   3 eggs

Instructions

   Preheat oven to 350° F.

   Combine all ingredients in a bowl and mix thoroughly. Roll into 1 ½" balls and place on a baking sheet. Bake for 18-20 minutes.

   This makes around fifty to sixty meatballs.

Broccoli and Cheese Quiche

Ingredients

10 oz. broccoli

¾ cup shredded mozzarella cheese

3 slices of lean ham

5 eggs

1 cup of sliced mushrooms

Instructions

Spray a pan with cooking spray.

Layer the pan with mushrooms, chopped broccoli, cheese and ham.

Beat eggs with water then pour in pan.

Bake at 350° F for twenty minutes.

Serves 6.

Egg Crepes

Ingredients

2 eggs

2 tbsp heavy cream

Instructions

Blend the ingredients in a blender.

Heat a pan with some oil.

Pour the mixture in the pan and as it starts to come away from the edges, turn carefully with a spatula. Slide the crepe onto a place until the mixture is finished.

Season with cinnamon and artificial sweetener.

Serves 1.

Hash Brown Potato Cakes

Ingredients

   1 lb round red potatoes

   1 tbsp olive oil

   ½ onion, thinly sliced

   ¼ tsp salt

   2 tsp fresh thyme

   Nonstick cooking spray

   1/8 tsp black pepper, ground

Instructions

Preheat oven to 300 degrees F. Peel and shred potatoes, rinse with cold water, drain well, pressing lightly then pat dry with paper towels and put in a large bowl. Stir onion, thyme, salt, oil, and pepper into the potatoes.

Coat a nonstick saucepan with cooking spray. Preheat the skillet over medium-high heat. For every cake, scoop a tablespoon of the potato mixture onto the skillet. Press down the potato mixture with a spatula to flatten evenly. Cook for five minutes then turn the potatoes and cook for another five minutes or until golden brown.

Place the cooked potatoes on a baking sheet. Keep them warm and uncovered in the oven as you cook the remaining potato cakes.

Serves 8.

Low carb Main dishes

Steak with garlic butter

Ingredients

    4 lb beef sirloin steak

    2 tsp garlic powder

    ½-cup butter

    4 cloves garlic, minced

    Black pepper and salt to taste

Instructions

Prepare an outdoor grill for high heat.

In a small pan, over medium heat, melt the butter and cook the garlic then set aside.

Grill the steaks for five minutes each side. Once done, transfer to warmed plates and brush the tops with the garlic butter. Allow to rest for around two minutes before serving.

Chicken breasts stuffed with spinach

Ingredients

    4 skinless, boneless chicken breasts

    1 10 oz. package chopped spinach, thawed and drained

    2 cloves garlic, chopped

    ½ cup crumbled feta cheese

    ½ cup mayonnaise

    4 slices of bacon

Instructions

    Preheat oven to 375 degrees F.

    Mix the mayonnaise, feta cheese, spinach and garlic until well blended then put aside.

    Butterfly the chicken wings ensuring not to cut all the way through.

    Spoon the spinach mixture into the chicken breasts and wrap each with a piece of bacon then secure using a toothpick. Put in a shallow baking dish and cover.

    Bake for one hour or until the chicken is no longer pink.

Serves 4.

Braised Balsamic Chicken

Ingredients

  6 skinless, boneless chicken breast halves

  ½ cup balsamic vinegar

  2 tbsp olive oil

  1 tsp garlic salt

  1 onion, sliced

  Ground black pepper to taste

  ½ tsp dried thyme

  1 cup of diced tomatoes

  1 tsp dried oregano

  1 tsp dried basil

  1 tsp dried rosemary

Instructions

Season the chicken with the garlic salt and pepper.

Heat oil in a pan over medium heat, cook the chicken until browned for around three to four minutes each side. Add the onions and cook until the onions have browned.

Pour the diced tomatoes and the vinegar over the chicken, season with oregano, thyme, rosemary and basil. Simmer the chicken for twenty-five minutes or until the juices run clear. This should be around 15 minutes.

Serves 6.

Honey Mustard Pork burgers

Ingredients

    1 lb ground pork breakfast sausage

    1 egg white, whisked

    1 cup plantain chips

    1 garlic clove, minced

    3 tbsp bacon fat

    1/2tsp garlic powder

    Black pepper and salt to taste

    1 tbsp raw honey

    1 avocado, sliced

    1 tsp yellow mustard

    1 tsp Dijon mustard

    Arugula to garnish

Instructions

Preheat the oven to 350 degrees F.

Put the plantain chips in the food processor and pulse until broken down into breadcrumb consistency.

Place the egg white in one bowl and the plantain crumbs in another. Dip each burger patty in the egg whites then plantain mixture to coat burgers completely then sprinkle with salt, garlic powder and pepper.

Heat a cast iron skillet over medium high heat, place two tbsp of bacon fat in the skillet and add the minced garlic.

Immediately the garlic becomes fragrant, add the pork burgers to the pan and cook both sides for four minutes.

Once the burgers are cooked on each side, place in the oven and cook for ten minutes. .

Whisk together the mustards, honey, and slice up the avocado.

Remove the burgers from the oven and allow them to rest for three minutes to prevent the juices from coming out.

Top each burger with the avocado and honey mustard.

Serves 4.

Herb crusted Salmon

Ingredients

- 2 salmon fillets

- 2 tbsp fresh parsley

- 1 tbsp coconut flour

- 1 tbsp Dijon mustard

- 2 tbsp olive oil

- 2 cups arugula

- Juice of 1 lemon

- ¼ red onion, sliced

- 1 tbsp white wine vinegar

- Black pepper and salt to taste

Instructions

Preheat oven to 450 degrees F.

Place the salmon on a baking sheet lined with foil.

Top the salmon with Dijon mustard and 1 tablespoon olive oil and rub into the salmon.

Mix the coconut flour, salt, pepper and parsley.

Sprinkle the toppings on the salmon then pat into the salmon using your hand.

Place in the oven for ten to 15 minutes.

While the salmon is cooking, mix the arugula, onion, lemon juice, salt, pepper, white wine vinegar and 1 tablespoon of olive oil.

Once cooked, top the salmon with the salad.

Low carb soups and salads

Bacon and Chicken Soup

Ingredients

12 slices bacon

10 oz. boneless skinless cooked chicken breasts

1 onion, diced

1 cup heavy whipping cream

1 bell pepper, chopped

1 cup chicken broth

1 1/3 cup Mexican shredded cheese

10 oz. cream cheese

8 celery stalks

1 yellow squash

1 small zucchini squash

8 cups of water

Instructions

Allow the water to boil and add any seasonings you want.

Chop all vegetables and add to the pot then reduce heat and allow to simmer.

Fry the bacon until crisp and set aside.

Chop the chicken into cubes, fry until crisp and put aside. Crunch the bacon into small pieces.

Add the chicken broth and cream. Simmer for twenty minutes.

Serve and top with Mexican cheese, bacon and cream cheese.

Tomato soup

Ingredients

28 ounce can diced tomatoes, undrained

2 cups chicken, broth

½ cup onion

2 tbsp butter

1 cup heavy cream

2 tbsp parsley, minced

Black pepper and salt to taste

Instructions

Sauté onion in butter until tender. Add the tomatoes with their liquid and broth then bring to a boil. Simmer for five minutes. Puree using a stick blender until you achieve a smooth consistency.

Stir in the cream and adjust the seasoning. Stir in the parsley and serve immediately.

Makes 6-8 servings or six cups.

Cream of Asparagus Soup

Ingredients

2 lb asparagus

2 tbsp low fat sour cream

6 cups fat free chicken broth

1 tbsp butter

1 medium onion, chopped

Salt and pepper to taste.

Instructions

Melt the butter on a large pot over low heat. Add onion and sauté on low heat for around 2 to 3 minutes.

Snap off the tough ends of the asparagus and discard. Chop the asparagus in two-inch pieces and add to the pot. Add the chicken broth, pepper and salt. Cover and cook for around 20-25 minutes.

Remove from the heat, add the sour cream, and puree until smooth using a hand held mixer.

Shrimp and Avocado Salad

Ingredients

Marinade

3 tbsp limejuice

½ cup chopped fresh cilantro

2 tbsp extra virgin olive oil

1/8 tsp fresh black pepper

Salt to taste

Salad

4 cups lettuce

2 ripe avocados

1 lb cooked shrimp, deveined and tail removed

Instructions

Pour the marinade over the shrimp, stir to coat and allow it to refrigerate for around an hour.

Wash and dry the lettuce and divide among plates.

Cut the avocado into wedges and sprinkle over the lettuce.

Top with the marinated shrimp and the leftover dressing.

Serves 4. If taken as dinner, serves 2.

Enchilada Chicken Avocado Salad

Ingredients

    1 cup of leftover chicken

    ½ Avocado, diced

    1 mango, peeled and diced

    1 small head of hearts of romaine, shredded.

Instructions

    Chop the romaine. Place the enchilada chicken on top.

    Add the avocado and mongo on top of that.

Serves two.

Cucumber Salad

Ingredients

1 ½ English Cucumbers

1 tsp salt

2 tbsp cilantro, Chopped

4 large green onions

¼ cup fresh lemon juice

1 tsp lemon zest

¼ cup extra virgin olive oil

1/8 tsp freshly cracked pepper.

Instructions

Slice the cucumbers finely. Sprinkle with salt and allow them to sit on a colander in the sink for an hour.

Rinse the cucumbers thoroughly and let them drain on paper towels.

Slice green onions, chop the cilantro and zest the lemon. Combine these three with lemon juice, cracked pepper and olive oil.

Pour the dressing over the cucumber and mix thoroughly.

Apple Zucchini Crisp

Ingredients

1 cup of apples, peeled and sliced

2 cups of zucchini, peeled halved and sliced thinly

2 tsp cinnamon, divided

¼ cup splenda brown sugar

A pinch of nutmeg

3 tbsp lemon juice

1/3 cup sliced almonds

1/3 cup almond meal

1 tsp vanilla extract

1/3 cup chopped pecans

¼ cup butter melted

Instructions

Preheat oven to 375 degrees F.

Toss the zucchini, apples, lemon juice and one teaspoon of cinnamon powder.

Pour into a baking dish.

Mix the remaining one teaspoon of cinnamon, brown sugar, almond meal, nutmegs, pecans and almonds together.

Stir in the vanilla with melted butter and pour over the nut mixture while mixing thoroughly.

Crumble the nut mixture over the zucchini and apples.

Bake while uncovered for thirty minutes

Serves 8.

Conclusion

Thank you again for downloading this book!

I hope this book was able to help you understand what the low carb diet is all about what to eat sparingly and what to avoid. This is the first step towards losing weight using the low carb diet. It is important that you start adopting the diet gradually so as not to overwhelm yourself which can lead to your eventual failure. You can start by substituting one of your meals with a low carb meal and overtime start changing your diet slowly with your goal to be to live a low carb diet lifestyle for permanent weight loss.

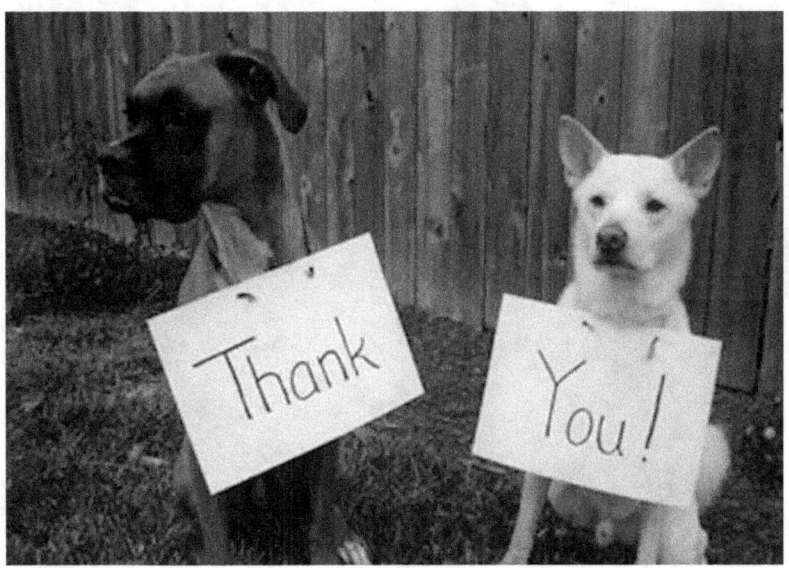

Finally, if you enjoyed this book, please take the time to share your thoughts and post a review on Amazon. It'd be greatly appreciated!

Thank you and good luck!

www.ingramcontent.com/pod-product-compliance
Lightning Source LLC
Chambersburg PA
CBHW061928280526
45787CB00004B/1525